Fertility

A Naturopathic Approach

Jane Semple, MA, ND

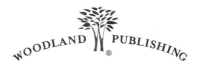

WOODLAND PUBLISHING

For permissions, ordering information, or bulk quantity discounts, contact: Woodland Publishing, 448 East 800 North, Orem, Utah 84097

Visit our Web site: www.woodlandpublishing.com
Toll-free number: (800) 777-2665

The information in this book is for educational purposes only and is not recommended as a means of diagnosing or treating an illness. All matters concerning physical and mental health should be supervised by a health practitioner knowledgeable in treating that particular condition. Neither the publisher nor the author directly or indirectly dispenses medical advice, nor do they prescribe any remedies or assume any responsibility for those who choose to treat themselves.

Cataloging-in-Publication data is available from the Library of Congress.

ISBN 978-1-58054-466-5

Printed in the United States of America

Contents

A couple is said to be infertile if pregnancy does not result after one year of normal sexual activity without contraceptives. About 25 percent of couples experience infertility at some point in their reproductive lives, with the incidence of infertility increasing with age. (CMDT, 2004) In 1964, infertility was estimated at 12 percent. (Cheraskin)

Although sources differ somewhat, when a couple is unable to conceive the husband is found to be infertile about one-third of the time; the wife one-third of the time; and no specific problem can be found for the remaining third. Most sources of infertility can be treated naturally.

In nature, animals reproduce until food becomes scarce, then fertility decreases. In this way, the population remains more stable and animals do not face mass starvation.

How does this relate to human fertility? After all, we are able to grow food to keep up with population increases. But, we are starving in a sea of plenty. Our over-farmed soil is lacking in nutrients, resulting in nutrient-deficient crops. Fast food, over-processed food and additives increase calories, while robbing foods of their nutritional value.

I am convinced the majority of human infertility is due to poor nutrition and lifestyle choices, which can be reversed. I have been treating infertility with naturopathic remedies for over a decade, and I have a wall of baby pictures to that they work.

Causes of Infertility

Female

Smoking, alcohol and recreational and pharmaceutical drugs have been cited as causes of reduced fertility in women. Hyper- or hypothyroid, overly rigorous exercise resulting in low sex hormones, obesity and excessive thinness and undernutrition resulting in vitamin deficiencies can reduce female fertility.

It is interesting that being excessively over- or underweight can interfere with fertility. Estrogens are produced by the ovaries, adrenals and in fat cells. Thus, too much or too little fat may disrupt the delicate hormone balance needed for conception and pregnancy.

Chronic vaginal infections, including yeast, interfere with the sperm's ability to survive in the vagina. Fallopian tubes may be scarred or blocked by endometrial tissue, and endometriosis and fibroid tumors in the uterus also reduce the ability of a fertilized egg to implant. All of these conditions respond well to herbal treatment. Fallopian tubes may become obstructed, interfering with conception. Blockage by endometrial tissue can usually be corrected herbally, but may require surgery.

The sperm simply delivers the paternal chromosomes to the ovum at fertilization. The ovum must provide the nourishment and genetic programming to support the embryonic development for nearly a week after conception. The blastocyst (preembryo) moves through the fallopian tube and must implant in the uterus.

The blastocyst attaches to the endometrial tissue and literally eats its way in. Endometriosis and fibroid tumors can interfere with implantation by not providing a hospitable surface for the blastocyst to attach. On the other hand, low estrogen levels can reduce the thickness of the endometrial lining to such an extent that the blastocyst cannot burrow deep enough to hang on.

If you have not already been counseled about determining when you're most fertile, I suggest that you consult *Women's Bodies, Women's Wisdom* by Christiane Northrup, MD. Dr. Northrup offers an excellent description of determining ovulation through cervical mucus discharge. Cervical mucus is rich in estrogen during the time a woman is fertile. Estrogen-rich mucus contains channels that assist the sperm in swimming to their destination.

Male

Semen analysis is performed to assess male fertility. A sample is donated after a period of sexual abstinence. The tests include:

- Volume: Normal ejaculate volume is 2 to 5 ml. Low volume may indicate a problem with the prostate gland or seminal vesicles.

- Sperm Count: Count may be reported per milliliter or as a total. Total spermatozoa per ejaculate commonly ranges from 60 to 100 million, or a minimum of 20 to 30 million, per milliliter. A low sperm count may reflect inflammation of the ductus deferens, the epididymis or prostate gland, or deficiencies due to suboptimal nutrition.

- Motility: Assessment of the sperm's swimming ability. A woman's cervical mucus assists the sperm during her fertile times.

- Morphology: Assessment of shape.

- Liquefaction: After ejaculation, semen coagulates and then liquefies after 15 to 30 minutes. Improper liquefaction time may indicate a problem with gland secretions.

Cigarettes, alcohol and recreational and pharmaceutical drugs, including antacids and pesticides, that mimic estrogen, negatively affect male fertility. Undernutrition resulting in a lack of vitamins and minerals reduces the quantity and quality of sperm production. Hyper- and hypothyroid may reduce sperm counts.

Many men are surprised to learn that antacids including cimetidine (Tagamet) and ranitidine (Zantac) may lead to infertility and impotence. The *Physician's Drug Handbook* also lists gynecomastia (male breast enlargement) as a potential adverse reaction if Tagamet is used for more than one month. It is best to work on digestive issues with a professional—your natural health-care practitioner.

Much has been written about decreasing sperm counts. When I first started treating infertility about 15 years ago, 60 million sperm per ejaculate was considered infertile; 60 million is now considered within the norm. Estimates vary, but I have seen reports stating that sperm counts have dropped by 40 to 50 percent since 1940. Despite the large number of studies conducted in many parts of the world, no consensus has been reached as to why sperm counts are dropping.

Sperm counts are highest for a man in his teens and twenties, dropping significantly during his thirties. A woman in her forties will have an easier time getting pregnant if her husband is five years younger rather than five years older.

Varicocele (enlargement of the veins of the spermatic cord) may reduce sperm production. Ejaculatory ducts may become obstructed.

Excessive heat can reduce sperm count. Men should avoid hot showers, saunas and hot tubs if they are trying to father a child. Also, many experts recommend that men wear boxer shorts, avoiding tight underwear and athletic supporters.

I once counseled a couple where the husband had a total sperm count near 20 million, just one-third of the minimum required to fertilize an egg. After a few months on my recommended program, his wife became pregnant. She then became pregnant a second time. I don't know what his sperm count was, since I don't do the testing. Nutritional supplements may have helped increase his sperm count or improved motility, either way—it worked.

Even when a man's sperm count is adequate, there is no guarantee he can father a child or that childlessness is due to an undiagnosed problem with his wife. A problem with any of the sperm characteristics listed above can reduce a man's ability to father a child.

A friend who practices acupuncture lists in her marketing brochure that she can treat infertility with acupuncture. At that time, I had a client with blocked fallopian tubes caused by an untreated sexually transmitted disease that she contracted when she was a teenager. I asked the acupuncturist if she had any success in treating blocked tubes, and she said that she hadn't had much success. I asked her how she treats her clients; she mentioned several things, all involving the wife. I said, "I can tell you why you're not having success, you're treating the wrong person. Treat the husband and they will get pregnant."

Even if a man's sperm count is within the norm, I insist he take nutritional supplements. I counseled a couple who could not become pregnant, even after three or four months of the wife doing a full supplement and nutrition program. The husband refused to take anything even though his sperm count was minimal (60 million) with low motility. In frustration, I suggested she find a sperm donor in the neighborhood bar—which would not be difficult. The husband got irritated and agreed to a minimal supplement program. They became pregnant within two months. Please understand that the husband was sitting in on the consultation, and I didn't really expect his wife to agree to have unprotected sex with a stranger. I got the result I wanted, and the husband agreed to take nutritional supplements, resulting in pregnancy.

Why does it take 60 million sperm to fertilize one egg? Because not one will stop and ask for directions. I made this joke up about fifteen years ago and one of my students put it on the Internet.

Conventional Medical Treatments

Some infertility problems require conventional medical intervention. These cases are rare, but they do occur. When conventional medical treatment is needed, it is usually to clear an obstruction with a surgical procedure.

One client came to me for a consultation after her initial appointment with a conventional medical fertility specialist. The specialist spent the entire time grilling the client on her husband's job, income, their savings, etc. My client did not understand why she was not examined or asked for her medical history. I explained that treating infertility is very expensive and is not covered by insurance. Before the medical doctor spent much time with her, she wanted to be sure the couple could afford her services.

Surgery

In women, obstruction of uterine tubes may benefit from microsurgery or require in vitro fertilization. In men with varicocele (enlargement of the veins of the spermatic cord), sperm characteristics often improve following surgical treatment. Obstruction of the ejaculatory ducts may also require surgical intervention. (CMDT)

Pharmaceutical Drugs

According to the *Physician's Drug Handbook* two drugs are approved for use in infertility. Clomiphene (also called Clomid, Milophene, and Serophene) is classified as an ovulation stimulant, though it is approved to treat both female and male infertility.

Adverse reactions include headache, blurred vision, photophobia (sounds like fear of having your picture taken, but it's actually light sensitivity), bloating, abdominal distension, nausea and vomiting. The scary ones are abnormal uterine bleeding, ovarian enlargement, cyst formation and breast discomfort.

Clomiphene promotes release of stimulating hormones that increase estrogens (estrone and estradiol). Estrogens promote follicle maturation and trigger ovulation.

Although the rate of ovulation following treatment is high, painful ovarian cysts form in 8 percent of patients, requiring that treatment be discontinued. Studies suggest a two- to threefold increased risk of ovarian cancer with the use of clomiphene for more than one year. (CMDT)

Bromocriptine/Parlodel is also approved for female fertility. It is an ergot alkaloid used to enhance dopamine receptors in Parkinson disease. Adverse reactions include delusions, depression, dizziness, drowsiness, fatigue, headache, insomnia, lightheadedness, mania, nervousness, seizures, heart attack, low blood pressure, blurred vision, nasal congestion, abdominal cramps, urinary frequency or retention and liver damage. Bromocriptine is derived from ergot, a fungus that grows on rye bread.

Alternative Treatments

Before spending time and money on invasive, expensive and possibly dangerous intervention, try some alternatives for a year. This includes improving your health with diet, lifestyle changes and by taking nutritional supplements. In the 1920s and 1930s research about the effects of vitamin supplements on fertility and infant health was in vogue. When Hitler came into power with his research into developing a "master race," there was a backlash. Some citizens claimed that giving vitamin supplements to women in the hopes of improving infant health and IQ was playing God. It's a shame that such ignorance caused thousands of birth defects and infant deaths every year. It is a shame that we are not as healthy as we could have been if physicians had been more aware of supplement research and passed this knowledge on to our mothers.

It is now accepted that supplementing may allow us to offset some of the negative effects of poor food choices and overprocessed foods. Armed with this knowledge, we can be healthier—and healthier parents create healthier children.

In 1937, a deficiency of folic acid was called the "universal teratogen" (causing birth defects). (Perlstein) It took 60 years for the U.S. government to require that folic acid be added back into grain products after it was processed out. Imagine how many birth defects and stillborn babies have resulted from this 60-year lapse.

There is no guarantee that you will conceive after a year of improved diet and supplementation. But even if you do eventually require conventional medical intervention, your body will be in better condition for parenting. Both you and your baby will benefit.

Diet and Supplement Research

In 1952, Dr. Jay Rommer stated: "Since nothing can come out of a human being except from what goes into him, one must assume a close correlation between food and fertility."

Observations regarding degenerative changes in the seminiferous tubules, atrophy of the testes and defective sperm production have been noted in various male animals. Similar findings have also been reported in female lower animals. These have been ascribed to a deficiency or an excess of various dietary factors and cited as evidence of fertility. (Cheraskin)

It is easier to manipulate fertility of lab animals. Infertility or reduced fertility has been induced with excess alcohol, sugar (20 percent of diet), low protein, fat deficiency or excess fat and vitamin A, vitamin E and calcium deficiencies.

Multiple studies offer a general consensus that diet and infertility are related. Human male and female infertility has been shown to be correlated with severe undernutrition, obesity, protein deficiency, as well as deficiency of various B vitamins, vitamin A, vitamin C, and vitamin E. Low zinc is related to reduced sperm production in men. In both men and women, fertility has been improved with supplementation. Fertility has also been correlated to both the quantity and the quality of protein intake, for both men and women. (Kennedy, 1926)

Thirty infertile men were given vitamin C at 1,000 mg, 200 mg, or a placebo. After one week, sperm count increased 140 percent in the 1,000 mg group, 112 percent in the 200 mg group, with no change in the placebo group. The 1,000 mg group also showed more improvement in sperm viability, motility, agglutination and abnormalities compared to the 200 mg group, with no change in the placebo group. However, both supplemented groups were nearly equal in all measures after 60 days. (Dawson, 1987) This suggests benefit from even moderate supplementation.

One study included 42 women who were not responsive to clomiphene, the pharmaceutical drug used to stimulate ovulation. Menses and ovulation were induced in 17 of the women with the addition of just 400 mg daily of vitamin C. (Igarashi, 1977)

Cervical infections are associated with infertility in women. In one study, cervical block (infection interfering with passage of sperm) was resolved in 9 of 14 women by eliminating sugar from the diet. In a second larger study, 47 of 65 cervical blocks resolved with sugar elimination. (Barton and Wiesner, 1948) I assume yeast or another organism that feeds on sugar was causing the infection. These organisms respond very well to diet changes, probiotics and herbal treatments.

Administration of 200 mg of vitamin E daily to 55 males with low sperm counts and sperm abnormalities produced an immediate increase in sperm count with some improvement in motility and a reduction of abnormal sperm. Of the 55 men, 20 had their semen value increase to normal and an additional 21 showed marked improvement. (Linder, 1958)

A zinc deficiency is associated with decreased sperm count, motility and low testosterone levels. (Skandhan, 1978; Abbasi, 1980; Mbtizvo, 1987)

In addition to infertility, poor-quality diets, low protein (below 54 g per day) and vitamin deficiencies cause premature babies, stillborn and neonatal deaths, preeclampsia, toxemia, and maternal death. If you are interested in further study, I recommend Dr. E. Cheraskin's book *Diet and Disease.*

Recommendations

Diet

I've been recommending diet and nutritional supplements to infertile couples for over a decade, and I have a wall of baby pictures to prove that this approach works.

Get rid of junk food, processed food, excess sugar, soda pop and other empty calories. Eat organic vegetables and fruit abundantly. I consider corn and potatoes to be grains, not vegetables. Keep grains and starches within reason. Eat free-range, hormone-free meat. If you do not consider yourself to be sufficiently informed on diet issues, please see a naturopath or other natural health-care practitioner for specific recommendations.

Since the father contributes 50 percent of the DNA, diet and supplementation is important prior to conception. His support is important in helping the mother stay with her healthy diet through the gestational and breastfeeding period.

I recommend the mother eat sufficient animal protein. This is important for fertility, a healthy pregnancy and a healthy baby. Various studies have tested protein intake between 90 g and 120 g daily with excellent results. (Cheraskin) I have seen two women who became vegetarians because they thought it was healthy, but they had both physically and mentally challenged babies.

I recommend that both parents follow Dr. Peter D'Adamo's *Eat Right for Your Type* diet, which is based on an individual's blood type, paying particular attention to meat and grains. I suggest that the mother-to-be take into consideration both her blood type and her husband's blood type, as both are an indication of what the baby's blood type will be.

Hydrotherapy

Ancient civilizations employed water in treatment of disease. These included Egyptians, Greeks, Romans, Persians, Hindus, Japanese and I am sure many more.

Cool or cold water contracts the blood vessels and tenses the muscles. Warm water opens the blood vessels, relaxes the muscles and promotes removal of impurities through the skin. I suggest alternating cool and warm over the abdominal area to increase circulation to the sex organs.

Increasing circulation will help to revitalize the sex organs.

You can alternate warm and cool in the shower. If you object to the shock to your system of the varying temperature on your entire body, I suggest sitting in a bath with a few inches of warm water. Alternate pouring cool, then warm, water from a half-gallon pitcher on your abdomen. How cool and how warm? I leave that entirely up to you.

Women should not do this during their menstrual cycle, especially if they tend toward cramping. Cool water can intensify muscle cramps.

Relaxation and Meditation

Stress can interfere with hormone production. Take time out of your day to relax a bit. Consider a relaxation CD or quiet music. I consider walking at a leisurely pace to be relaxing.

When a couple calls for a fertility consultation, my receptionist used to insist that the husband and wife come in together for the appointment. We could not believe how difficult this was due to schedule conflicts. I now agree to see either the husband or wife, then prepare recommendations for both.

You do need to get together at some time—you understand that, right?

Supplements

Women

Naturopathic medicine is about bringing the body back to a healthy state by using natural methods. We want to nudge the body into a state of homeostasis, a relatively constant internal environment. For women, this means a gentle rhythm of hormones, as nature intended. If a woman has any health issues, I suggest that we work on those for three to six months before she tries to become pregnant.

I'm discussing supplements last for a reason. If you skipped to this section to see what supplements you need to take to become pregnant, please go back and read the first part of the book first. The term *supplement* means "in addition," and using supplements along with a good diet can result in a healthy mom, a healthy pregnancy and a healthy baby.

I am very conservative about the supplements I recommend for someone who is actively trying to become pregnant. For example, I do not recommend a colon cleanse, a liver cleanse or other detox formulas for someone who is currently trying to conceive. I prefer that a woman do some cleansing and improve her general health for a few months, then try to conceive. A healthy mother has a better chance of having a healthy pregnancy and a healthy baby.

One client was in such a hurry to have a baby that she would not detox and build up her own health for a few months. She did not become pregnant despite trying for an entire year. The client and her husband decided she needed to work on her health and stopped trying to conceive and started adoption proceedings. After taking a few months to cleanse, detox and build her immune system, she became pregnant and now has a healthy baby girl.

If a woman is in good health and does not have a major identifiable problem, I start with a basic program, which consists of four supplements.

Prenatal vitamins: The one I recommend includes 800 mcg of folic acid with a B-complex and vitamins A, C, D and E with minerals. Be careful of prescription prenatal vitamins, as they are usually synthetic. A prenatal vitamin should not make you nauseous or cause constipation or diarrhea.

Calcium and Magnesium: Calcium (400 to 600 mg), magnesium (200 to 300 mg) with vitamin D and trace minerals. This amount of calcium should be sufficient if you're eating well. RDAs are based on calcium carbonate, which isn't highly absorbable. I use a combination calcium phosphate and calcium citrate with vitamin D and trace minerals, so lower doses are sufficient.

Red raspberry as a tea or capsule. Be sure you are getting a high-quality product. Follow the instructions on the package or the instructions of your naturopath or health-care practitioner. I also use red raspberry for clients at risk of miscarriage and recommend a moderate dose throughout pregnancy and breastfeeding.

Three of my clients have stopped a miscarriage by taking red raspberry. All three were able to carry their baby to full term.

Essential fatty acids like those contained in borage, black currant, evening primrose
and flaxseed oils. Fatty acids aid glandular function and enrich breast milk. A shortage of this nutrient is blamed for postpartum depression, so I recommend you continue taking this supplement throughout pregnancy and breastfeeding.

Several midwives have recommended that patients insert a caplet of evening primrose oil vaginally to soften the cervix three weeks before delivery. It is said to make delivery easier. I often wonder if during hard labor a woman isn't thinking, "This is easier!"

If a woman is not menstruating or ovulating regularly I suggest a wild yam and chaste tree (Vitex) combination. Several clients near the age of 45 became pregnant, with younger husbands, after ovulation became more regular with this combination.

Other Female Herbs

There are few studies on herbs used in fertility, so we have to depend on what has worked for us and others in the past. Your naturopath or herbalist may recommend some of the following herbs to promote pregnancy. Do not continue these herbs during pregnancy unless specifically recommended by a qualified naturopath or herbalist.

Chaste tree berry (Vitex) is used to tone and strengthen the tissue and organs of the female reproductive system. In 1943, Probst and Roth found that this plant has the ability to increase production of luteinizing hormone (LH), which stimulates the production of progesterone and acts like a mild or phyto-progesterone.

Chaste tree berry may be used to restore the body's balance after taking birth control pills for a period of time. Chaste tree should especially be considered with established luteal phase defect and high prolactin levels. Zinc and vitamin B6 (with a B-complex) may assist in regulating prolactin levels, though I could not find specific research. I recommend it in combination with wild yam for women who are not ovulating regularly.

Damiana is accepted by Germany's Commission E for use as an aphrodisiac and for treatment of sexual disorders. Damiana is considered a sexual restorative and tonic for the nervous and reproductive system. I have not used this herb for fertility, though other herbalists have recommended it in fertility combinations.

Dong quai is called the "queen of herbs," and it promotes blood flow to the reproductive organs and enhances fertility. This herb seems to have a mild estrogenic effect on the body. The noted herbalist Rosemary Gladstar recommends dong quai in her fertility tonic. Dong quai is highly prized by Asian herbal practitioners. It is not recommended for use during pregnancy and should be discontinued after a positive pregnancy test.

Iron levels should be checked. If your levels are low, your natural health practitioner may suggest a supplement to bring your levels up to normal. I do not recommend an inorganic iron supplement, such as one you would purchase from a drugstore. I use an herbal combination with red beet root, yellow dock root, red raspberry leaves, burdock and nettle.

Kelp: If a woman has a personal or family history of thyroid problems, I suggest a small dose of kelp. My hope is that the kelp will reduce the chances of passing on a weak thyroid and provide sufficient hormone to avoid birth problems related to thyroid. Kelp may be taken throughout your pregnancy.

Maca grows in the Peruvian highlands and is highly revered for its energy and libido-enhancing properties. South American herbalists have used maca for thousands of years to improve physical stamina, fertility and hormone balance.

Maca is used to enhance fertility in both men and women, with many anecdotal reports from naturopaths and herbalists. This herb is also used to enhance adrenal function and improve response to stress.

Probiotics are the good bacteria in the intestine. They include *Bifidobacterium bifidus, Bifidobacterium longum, Lactobacillus acidophilus, Lactobacillus rhamnosus, Lactobacillus casei* and many others. Probiotics keep the intestinal flora healthy, keeping yeast and "bad" bacteria under control. Your natural health practitioner may recommend a combination for use throughout pregnancy and breast-feeding.

Vitamin E at 400 IU daily is considered the fertility vitamin, though fertility is likely reduced with a severe shortage of any vitamin. I consider it optional for my clients who are eating well and have not been trying to conceive for very long. I add vitamin E for both husband and wife if there is no pregnancy after three to six months.

Wild yam root contains a phytoestrogen (plant estrogen) and the steroid diosgenin, which is a precursor to progesterone. Plants are self-contained systems that produce hormone-like substances for their own use. Plant estrogens are not as "large" or as active as human hormones. These estrogen-like substances promote beneficial effects on the female glandular system by occupying cell hormone receptor sites.

Native American women often consumed wild yam root as a form of birth control. The herb does not interfere with normal ovulation or menses but is thought to make a woman's egg resistant to fertilization.

I sometimes recommend a small temporary dose of wild yam with chaste tree to stimulate menses and ovulation for a few months. I have found it especially helpful for women over the age of 40, as the two seem to promote appropriate hormone cycles. I recommend that my clients stop taking wild yam after they become pregnant, but the herbalist John Christopher, ND, recommended it through pregnancy as a uterine tonic.

Supplements
Male

It takes about nine weeks to produce sperm cells (spermatogenesis). This suggests that in a little over two months of healthy eating and supplementation, a man can pass on healthier genes. Men are not usually good at taking pills, so I keep my recommendation to a minimum. I suggest three to four supplements to be taken at least until conception. Some men feel so much better on the supplements that they continue taking them.

Multiple vitamins that include a high-dose B-complex, antioxidants and minerals. The B-complex portion of the vitamin is especially important in producing sperm with a solid DNA structure.

Zinc is essential for tissue growth, maintenance and repair, as well as the functions of more than 200 human enzymes, including those necessary for DNA and RNA synthesis. It is a building block of cell membranes.

Zinc aids in reproductive organ function, especially the prostate, and is needed to increase sperm production and increase potency and sex drive. The multiple I recommend contains 15 mg, then I add an additional supplement with 25 mg to 50 mg per day.

Wild American ginseng has accumulated much folklore regarding its uses. It has been used to increase stamina, vitality and physical performance. Wild roots are said to have a slightly higher potency compared to the farmed variety.

The root of ginseng resembles a human figure. Medical herbalists in many ancient societies presumed a plant's appearance contained clues to its medicinal uses. Ancient herbalists believed a divine being placed herbs on earth for our use and left clues as to the herb's uses. In European herbalism this became known as the doctrine of signatures. Thus, the formation of the ginseng root indicates that it is a whole-body tonic.

In Europe, ginseng from Asia was highly prized for centuries. A Jesuit living among the Iroquois near Montreal discovered American ginseng in the early 18th century. Ginseng brought such an outrageous price in Europe, it was like finding gold.

As with other rare herbs, be sure you are purchasing from a reputable supplier. Several organizations have tested commercial ginseng products and found no trace of ginseng. If the price looks too good to be true, it probably is. If you cannot afford wild American ginseng, you may substitute Siberian ginseng, now commonly called eleuthero.

Wild American ginseng should be taken with caution if you have a history of high blood pressure. If you take ginseng, please keep track of blood pressure and discontinue if the herb raises it. Consider taking eleuthero, as it does not commonly have the effect of raising blood pressure.

Some of my clients come to me after they have had fertility counseling with a conventional medical doctor, so some men have already had a semen analysis. One client had a sperm count of 20 million per milliliter, which climbed to 37 million after a few months on my recommended supplements. His physician agreed that the supplements might have helped. Yes—we will gladly take credit.

Other Male Herbs

As with female herbs, there are few scientific studies on herbs used to increase fertility in males. But there's no shortage of anecdotal reports. Your herbalist or naturopath may also recommend other herbs they have had good results with in the past.

Damiana contains alkaloids (chemical components) that suggest it has a mild testosterone-like action. This herb has been used historically as an aphrodisiac, circulatory stimulant, tonic and restorative. Damiana is said to rejuvenate the male sex organs, treating impotence and premature ejaculation. Damiana has a long history of use among South American natives.

Eleuthero is referred to as an adaptogen, a substance that corrects or normalizes bodily functions. It may assist with adrenal and thyroid functions as well. The Chinese have used eleuthero for over 2,000 years to increase longevity, vitality and general health. Eleuthero has been used to normalize adrenal, thyroid and pancreatic function and has also demonstrated antioxidant and immune-enhancing effects by assisting white blood cells.

American ginseng is not recommended for people with high blood pressure, but eleuthero is said to normalize blood pressure. If your pressure is particularly high, keep track of your it after starting this supplement to be sure it is not adversely effected. Eleuthero was formerly called Siberian ginseng, though it does not contain many of the alkaloids (chemical components) of true ginseng and is not botanically related to true ginseng. The producers of American ginseng became concerned that "Siberian ginseng"—which is not a ginseng at all—was cheaper than their product. Responding to this concern, the FDA required that manufacturers and distributors of Siberian ginseng discontinue using the word *ginseng* on product packaging and in marketing materials. Producers decided to use a portion of the Latin name—*Eleuthorococcus senticosus*—resulting in eleuthero.

Kelp: If a man has a personal or family history of thyroid problems, I suggest a small dose of kelp. I supplement blood tests with iridology, which determines strengths and weaknesses through analysis of the eye. A weak thyroid can reduce sperm counts.

L-arginine is an amino acid required for male fertility. It dilates the blood vessels, so it's helpful in regulating blood pressure and improving erectile dysfunction. L-arginine is abundant in meat and is also found in dark chocolate.

Anyone suffering from herpes (cold sores or genital) or other viruses should be cautious in taking supplemental 1-arginine. Work with your natural health-care practitioner in balancing 1-arginine with 1-lysine. Excessive 1-arginine may stimulate growth of viruses.

Maca is a highly prized South American herb used to increase energy and stamina. It is recommended as an aphrodisiac and to enhance fertility in both men and women. In men, maca is a treatment for impotence and erectile dysfunction.

A four-month study of nine men found that oral treatment with maca significantly increased semen volume, total sperm count and sperm motility. (Gonzales, 2001)

Sarsaparilla: If you watch old westerns you may recall a young man walking into the saloon and ordering sarsaparilla.

One of the old timers says, "Sarsaparilla, why that's a sissy drink." This herb does indeed promote testosterone production. In the past, young men used sarsaparilla to mature more quickly through puberty.

In adult men, sarsaparilla is said to sustain youth and sexual vigor. Two steroidal alkaloids found in this herb may act as precursors to cortisone and other steroidal hormones, like testosterone.

How to Locate a Practitioner

You may be able to conceive by following the suggestions in this book, especially if you do not have significant underlying conditions. If you feel you need additional guidance, please look for a natural health practitioner in your area. Ask how many years they have been practicing and how much experience they have dealing with fertility.

Check your local phone directory under Naturopaths, Herbs or Alternative Medicine. You may also contact the American Naturopathic Medical Association (ANMA), PO Box 96273, Las Vegas, NV 89193. The ANMA is the oldest and largest naturopathic association, with approximately 4,000 members. Ask for the name of two or three practitioners in your area, so that you can work with the person you feel most comfortable with.

I am very interested in your success stories. You may contact me by mail at Alternative Healing Institute, 4965 Dover Center Road, North Olmsted, OH 44070. If you wish to receive a reply, you must include a self-addressed stamped envelope.

Please send a picture of your baby. I'll put it on my wall.

Bibliography

Abbasi A., et al. "Experimental zinc deficiency in man: effect on testicular function." *Journal Laboratory Clinical Medicine* 96(3):544–50, 1980.

Anderson, R., et al. "Ethanol-induced male infertility: impairment of spermatozoa." *Journal of Pharmacological Experimental Therapies* 225(2):47, 1983.

Anderson, R., et al. "Male reproductive tract sensitivity of ethanol: a critical overview." *Pharmacological Biochemical Behavior* 1:30 5–10, 1983.

Barney, Paul, MD. *Doctor's Guide to Natural Medicine.* Pleasant Grove, UT: Woodland Publishing, 1998.

Barton, M. and Wiesner, B. P. "The role of special diets in the treatment of female infertility." *British Medical Journal,* 4584, 847–51, November 1948.

Cheraskin, E., W.M. Ringsdorf and J.W. Clark. *Diet and Disease,* New Canaan, CT: Keats Publishing, 1968, 88–102.

Christopher, John, ND. *School of Natural Healing.* Springville, UT: Christopher Publications, 1976.

Dawson, E. "Effect of ascorbic acid on male fertility." *Annals of the New York Academy of Sciences* 498:312–23, 1987.

Duke, James, PhD. *Green Pharmacy,* Emmaus, PA: Rodale Press, 1997.

Gladstar, Rosemary. *Herbal Healing for Women.* New York: Fireside Books, 1993.

Gonzales, G., et al. "Maca improved semen parameters in adult men." *Asian Journal of Andrology* 3(4):301–03, 2001.

Herb Allure Resource Toolkit, P. O. Box 1048, Jamestown, NY 14702, 2004.

Hoffman, David. *New Holistic Herbal.* Boston: Element Books, 1990.

Igarashi, M. "Augmentative effect of ascorbic acid upon induction of human ovulation in clomiphene-ineffective anovulatory women." *International Journal Fertility* 22:168–73, 1977.

Kennedy, W. "Diet and sterility." *Physician's Review,* 6:485–503, 1926.

Linder, E. "Therapeutics of Vitamin E in Spermatogenesis." *International Vitamin Forum* 29:33–40, 1958.

Mabey, Richard. *New Age Herbalist.* New York: Simon and Shuster, 1988.

Martini, F. *Fundamentals of Anatomy and Physiology.* Saddle River, NJ: Prentice Hall, 1995.

Mbtizvo, M., et al. "Seminal plasma zinc levels in fertile and infertile men." *South African Medical Journal* 71:266, 1987.

Meaker and Davis. *Gynecology and Obstetrics,* vol. 2. New York: W. F. Prior Company, 1964.

Mendleson, J. "Alcohol effects on reproductive function in women." *Psychiatry Letter* 4(7):35–38, 1986.

Northrup, Christiane, MD. *Women's Bodies, Women's Wisdom,* MD. New York: Bantam Books, 1998.

Perlstein & Levinson, "Birth weight: its statistical correlation with various factors." *American Journal Dis. Child,* June 1937.

Probst, V. and Roth, D., *German Medicine,* 204, 1943.

Reynolds and Macomber *Fertility and Sterility in Human Marriages.* Philadelphia: Saunders Company, 1924.

Rommer, J. *Sterility: Its Causes and Its Treatment.* Springfield: Charles Thomas Company, 1952.

Skandhan, K. "Semen electrolytes in normal and infertile subjects." *Experientia* 34:1476–77, 1978.

Tierney, Lawrence, Stephen McPhee and Maxine Papadakis. *Current Medical Diagnosis and Treatment* (CMDT). New York: McGraw-Hill, Medical Publishing Division, 2004.

Williams and Wilkins. *Physician's Drug Handbook,* 10th edition. New York: Lippincott, 2005.

About the Author

Dr. Jane Semple received her master's degree from Case Western Reserve, graduating first in her class in 1984. She completed a dual Doctorate in Naturopathy and Naturopathic Ministry from Trinity College of Natural Health. She has been an herbalist and naturopathic practitioner for twenty years.

Dr. Semple was a professor at Cuyahoga Community College for six years and Baldwin-Wallace College for three years. She developed an Anatomy and Physiology module for Trinity College of Natural Health.

She founded the Alternative Healing Institute to bring training for alternative therapies to individuals and medical professionals. She develops and teaches Continuing Education courses for those in the medical field.

Dr. Semple is an active member of the American Naturopathic Medical Association, the Association of Nutritional Consultants, American Botanical Council and Coalition for Natural Health. She is a Health Freedom advocate.

She has been listed in *Who's Who of American Women* since 1985, and *Who's Who in Medicine and Healthcare* since 2004. She was honored as a Woman of Achievement in Ohio in April 2005.

Other Books by the Author in the Woodland Health Series

Alzheimer Disease: A Naturopathic Approach

Blood Pressure: A Naturopathic Approach

Cholesterol and Inflammation: A Naturopathic Approach

HPV and Cervical Dysplasia: A Naturopathic Approach

Influenza: Epidemics, Pandemics and the Bird Flu

Parkinson Disease: A Naturopathic Approach